Exercise

The importance of exercise and its guides. Why you need exercise

By

Robert L. Sievert

Table of contents

1. Introduce,

2. What is exercise

3. What exercise burns the most calories

4. Are exercise bike good

5. Can exercise low blood pressure

6. Which exercise burns the most belly fats

7. Why regular exercise is important

8. Exercise without equipment

9. How exercise improves mental health

10. Exercise reduces stress

Introduction

Scientific training methods to live the last years of life more energetically, physically taller, and in better shape with simple weight training to improve endurance beyond 50 years old. As you age, your lean muscle begins to decline. Over time, this can lead to weakness, reduced physical ability, and the inevitable difficulty of performing activities of daily living as you enter your 60s or older. Loss of muscle mass can eventually lead to a lack of strength, stability, and balance, leading to an increased risk of falls, related injuries, and further physical impairment. But you can do something about it. Would you like to learn about the best exercises for seniors to build strength and increase performance later in life?

What is exercise

Exercise can be done for a variety of purposes, including to aid growth and improve strength, develop muscles and the cardiovascular system, honing athletic skills, lose or maintain weight, improve health, or just for fun.[2] In terms of health benefits, the recommended amount of exercise depends on the goal, the type of exercise, and the person's age. Aqua running and weight training are body activities that improve or maintain physical fitness as well as overall health and wellness. Physical activity is essential for maintaining physical fitness and can help maintain a healthy weight, regulate the digestive system, build and maintain healthy bone density, muscle strength, and joint mobility, promoting physiological well-being, reduce the risk of surgical procedures, and strengthen the immune system. Exercise may improve quality of life and life expectancy, according to some studies. The mortality rate of those who engage in moderate to vigorous physical activity is lower than that of those who are not physically active. The majority of the benefits of exercise are achieved with approximately 3500 metabolic equivalents (MET) minutes per week, with diminishing returns at higher levels of activity. For instance, climbing stairs for ten minutes, vacuuming for fifteen minutes, and gardening for twenty minutes are all examples of the benefits of exercise. Overall, physical inactivity accounts for 9% of premature mortality worldwide.

What exercise burns the most calories

The sport that burns the most calories per hour is running. Swimming, stationary biking, and jogging are all excellent alternatives. Additionally, HIIT exercises are excellent for calorie burning. Exercises that burn calories in a short amount of time At home Things to think about and how to get started If you want to burn the most calories for your money, you might want to start running. The most calories are burned per hour when running. However, if running isn't your thing, you can also burn calories by swimming, jumping rope, and doing HIIT workouts. Depending on your preferences and fitness level, you can perform any of these exercises in any order.

There are a number of factors that influence how many calories are burned, including: duration of exercise, intensity, pace, weight, and height. In general, the more weight you have, the more calories you will burn while exercising.

Work with a personal trainer to find out the exact number. During a workout, they can figure out how many calories you burn on your own.

The top 12 exercises that burn the most calories are listed in the table below. The most calories are burned per hour by these exercises. Keep in mind that the listed calories are an estimate. Your weight, intensity, and duration all play a role in determining how many calories you burn.

Swimming (casual) Jogging Hiking Running Water polo Bicycling Circuit training Jump rope Stationary bicycling Rowing machine Aerobic dance In a time crunch You can perform exercises that burn a lot of calories even if you don't have much time. The key is to concentrate on workouts with high intensity that quickly raise your heart rate.

One popular method is high-intensity interval training or HIIT. It involves exercising for short periods of time at more than 70% of your aerobic capacity.

Alternating between 30-second speed and 1-minute rest intervals is one HIIT method. In as little as 30 minutes, you can burn a lot of calories by engaging in high-intensity workouts.

If you're short on time, try these exercises to burn a lot of calories.

Running with your knees high Calories burned in 30 minutes: 240 to 355.5 is a vigorous cardio workout for high-knee running. It makes your heart beat faster and makes your lower body stronger. High-knee running, which is a high-intensity exercise, helps you burn calories quickly.

To perform this task:

While keeping your knees as high as possible, run in place.

Pump your arms quickly up and down.

In 30 minutes, calories burned from butt kicks:

Butt kicks, like high-knee running, are a cardio workout between 240 and 355.5. By doing high-intensity butt kicks, you can burn calories quickly in 30 minutes.

To perform this task:

Move one heel toward your buttocks.

With the other heel, do it again.

While pumping your arms, quickly alternate your heels.

Climbers of mountains Calories burned in 30 minutes: 240 to 355.5 The mountain climber is a cardio workout that also works the whole body. You'll burn a lot of calories quickly because you have to use your entire body.

To perform this task:
In the plank position, begin. Cover your hands with your shoulders. Work your core. Move your right knee in front of your chest. Back to the plank. Use your left knee to repeat.
Do so quickly.

Are exercise bikes good

1. Improves cardiovascular fitness Cycling is an excellent cardio activity.

Exercises that are aerobic or cardiovascular, like cycling, make your heart, lungs, and muscles stronger. Additionally, they enhance oxygen and blood circulation throughout your body. In turn, this has the potential to improve your health in a number of ways, including:

improved brain and memory, lower blood pressure, better sleep, better blood sugar control, a stronger immune system, better mood, less stress, and more energy can aid in weight loss Depending on the intensity of your workout and your body weight, a stationary bike workout can burn more than 600 calories per hour. As a result, indoor cycling is a great way to burn calories quickly.

The key to losing weight is burning more calories than you eat.

3. burns fat A high-intensity workout helps you burn calories and build strength, both of which can help you lose weight.

According to a Trusted Source study from 2010, indoor cycling and a low-calorie diet helped participants in the study lose weight and fat. Additionally, it was successful in lowering levels of triglycerides and cholesterol. For twelve weeks, the participants cycled for 45 minutes three times per week and ate 1,200 calories per day. 4. Offers a Low-Income Workout A low-impact workout that uses smooth movements to strengthen bones and joints without putting a lot of stress on them is a stationary bike workout. Because of this, it's a good exercise option for people who have joint problems or injuries.

Running, jogging, jumping, and other high-impact aerobic exercises can put a lot of stress on your hips, ankles, knees, and other joints.

A stationary bike is kinder to your joints because your feet don't lift off the pedals, but it still provides a challenging and effective workout.

5. Builds muscle in the legs and lower body Riding a stationary bike can help you build muscle in your legs and lower body, especially if you use more resistance.

Your quadriceps, hamstrings, and calves can all benefit from the pedaling motion. It can also strengthen your glutes, back, and core muscles.

You can work your shoulders, biceps, and triceps as well as your upper body if you ride a bicycle with handles.

6. allows for interval training allows you to alternate brief bouts of vigorous exercise with longer bouts of less vigorous exercise. You can burn more calories in a shorter amount of time and improve your cardio fitness with this kind of training.

You can exercise at low, medium, or high intensities on

stationary bikes because they allow for a variety of resistance levels. Because of this, an interval training workout would be ideal.

7. Safer than cycling on the road Cycling outside can be a great way to exercise, but there are risks like distracted drivers, uneven or slick roads, and poor visibility.

Additionally, it may be challenging to find the motivation to go outside when the weather is hot and humid or cold and wet. Even if it were safe, it might not be.

You don't have to worry about traffic, road conditions, or the weather when you ride indoors. Any time of year, you can exercise safely at a comfortable temperature.

Can exercise low blood pressure

The heart gets stronger with regular exercise. With a stronger heart, more blood can be pumped with less effort. As a result, less force is applied to the arteries. Blood pressure falls as a result. Additionally, regular exercise aids in weight maintenance. One important way to control blood pressure is to lose weight. Losing even 5 pounds (or 2.3 kilograms) can lower blood pressure in overweight people.

Regular exercise takes between one and three months to have an effect on blood pressure. The advantages only last as long as you exercise.

How often do you need to exercise?

At least 150 minutes of moderate aerobic activity or 75 minutes of vigorous aerobic activity, or a combination of the two, should be your goal each week. On most days of the week, aim for at least 30 minutes of aerobic exercise.

Start slowly if you have never exercised before. You can divide your aerobic workout into three sessions of ten minutes each. You get the same benefit from this as from a 30-minute session.

Aerobic activity is any activity that increases heart and breathing rates. Examples include:

Cycling, climbing stairs, dancing, gardening, mowing the lawn and raking the leaves, jogging, swimming, and walking are all forms of active sports that seem to have the greatest impact on heart health.

If you sit for a lot of time each day, try to take five to ten minutes of movement and stretching breaks every hour. Numerous chronic diseases, including high blood pressure, are linked to an inactive or sedentary lifestyle. Try going for a quick walk or simply going to the kitchen or break room to get a drink of water to get some exercise into your day. It might be helpful to set a reminder on your computer or phone. Before beginning an exercise program, it's sometimes best to talk to your doctor, especially if:

You have a chronic health condition like diabetes, heart disease, or lung disease; you have high cholesterol or high blood pressure; you have had a heart attack; you have a family history of heart-related problems before the age of 55 in men and 65 in women; you experience pain or discomfort in your chest, jaw, neck, or arms while exercising; you become dizzy while exercising; you smoke or recently quit

smoking; you are overweight or obese; you are unsure if you are in good health; you haven't been
Pain in the chest, neck, jaw, or arm, dizziness, or fainting, severe shortness of breath, or an irregular heartbeat

Which exercise burns the most belly fats

Before performing these exercises, warm up for ten minutes. Take a 10-second break after warming up your muscles, then begin the following exercises:

1. Lower abs, upper abs, glutes, hamstrings, and quadriceps can all be targeted with the lying leg raise exercise for losing belly fat.

How to Perform: Lie on a mat. With your palms flat on the

floor, place your thumbs under your hips. Engage your core as you lift your feet off the ground and look up at the ceiling. This is where you should start.

Bring both of your legs back down slowly after raising them to a 90-degree angle.

Re-raise your legs just before you touch the floor. Perform three 15-rep sets.

2. Lower abs, upper abs, glutes, hamstrings, and quadriceps are all targets of the leg in and out exercise for losing belly fat.

How to Perform a Mat Sit With your palms flat on the mat, place your hands behind you. Lean slightly back and raise your legs off the ground. This is where you should start.

Put your legs in a tuck. Bring your upper body close to your knees simultaneously. Return to where you started. Perform two 20-rep sets.

3. Scissor Kicks: Scissor kicks are a low-impact exercise that targets the lower, upper, hamstring, and quadriceps, as well as the lower and upper abs.

How to Perform: Lie on a mat. You should have your palms below your hips.

Take your legs, back, and head off the ground. This is where you should start.

Reduce your left foot. Lift your left leg and lower your right leg just as it reaches the floor.

To finish a set, do this 12 times. Perform three 12-rep sets. Before moving on to the next exercise, take a 20-second break. Crunches: Crunches are a great way to lose belly fat. Target: Lower and upper abs.

How to Perform Lie down on a mat with your feet flat on the floor and your knees bent. Each ear should have a thumb at the back. The remaining fingers should be used to hold the back of your head. Take your eyes off the ground. This is where you should start.

Start the exercise by curling up and using your head to try to reach your knees.

Return to where you started. While curling up, make sure to inhale and exhale simultaneously. Perform two 12-rep sets.

Ten episodes of Kneeling Ab Wheel

Leg raises for 10 reps and side plank hip lifts for 20 reps (10 on each side).

Plank - Hold for as long as possible Russian twists - 20 reps (10 per side) McGill sit-up - 20 reps (10 per side)

Why regular exercise is important

Regular physical activity is one of the most important things you can do for your health. Being physically active can help you manage your weight, improve your brain health, strengthen your bones and muscles, lower your disease risk, and make it easier to do things you normally do.

There are some health benefits for adults who sit less and engage in any amount of moderate-to-vigorous physical activity. Physical activity is one of only a few lifestyle choices that have such a significant impact on health.

Everyone can reap the health benefits of physical activity, regardless of age, ability, ethnicity, or body type.

1. Following a session of moderate-to-vigorous physical activity, brain health improves immediately. Children between the ages of 6 and 13 benefit, as do adults who experience fewer short-term feelings of anxiety. Your ability to learn, think clearly, and make sound

decisions can all benefit from regular physical activity as you get older. It can also help you sleep better and lower your risk of depression and anxiety.

prevalent cancers Adults with higher levels of physical activity have lower rates of the following cancers:

Endometrium Esophagus (adenocarcinoma) Kidney Lung Stomach (cardia and non-cardia adenocarcinoma) Bladder Breast Colon (proximal and distal)

exercise without equipment

The warm-up Before starting, warm up. Quick walking or jogging for five minutes will suffice. Afterward, stretch or foam roll to reduce soreness.

To create a challenging routine, combine five to six of these exercises:

1. Rotational jacks are a good way to start a workout and are a variation of the jumping jack. They will make your muscles

warm and raise your heart rate.

Directions:

Begin with a wide stance and supple knees. Your arms should be parallel to the ground and extended straight out from your sides.

Keep your arms straight and keep your head and neck still. Rotate your torso so that your right-hand touches the ground and hinge forward at the hips.

Jump together while resuming your starting position.

Jump back out with your feet immediately, pivot backward,

and rotate to the left, putting your hand on the ground.

Restart the process. Twist once more to the right as you join your feet.

For three sets, perform 12 to 15 reps.

2. Reach-under planks are a fundamental (but difficult!) exercise. exercise that benefits the entire body. The reach-under feature further targets your core.

Directions:

On your hands, assume a high plank position.

Make sure your lower back doesn't sag and your core is braced. You should have a neutral neck and spine.

Tap your left thigh with your fingers as you raise your right hand off the ground. Go back to a plank.

Tap your right thigh with your left hand as you do it again, then return to a plank position.

Complete three sets of 20 taps in total.

3. Step-ups: Doing step-ups will make your lower body burn. Additionally, they are

excellent for developing balance and stability.

Directions:

Step with your feet together or stand in front of a bench that is at least knee height.

With your right foot, step onto the bench by pushing through your heel and raising your left knee.

As you get off the bench, step backward with your left leg.

With your right leg, perform 10 to 15 repetitions, then switch to your left leg and perform 10 to 15 repetitions.

Finish three sets.

4. Mountain climbers When you can perform a few sets of mountain climbers, you don't need to use weights. Your muscles and lungs will be on fire as you support yourself with your own weight and the knee drive.

Directions:

Lie on a high plank with your arms outstretched.

Drive your right knee up toward your chest while engaging your core and remaining neutral in your spine and neck. Drive your left knee immediately up toward your chest after extending it.

Keep good form and go as fast as you can during the 30-second repetition.

Finish all three sets.

5. Plyometric exercises like squats and jumps are ones that force your muscles to work hard in a short amount of time. Squat jumps are a good illustration. With just a few sets of these, you can get a lot for your money. Warning: Because of their high impact, you should proceed with

caution if your joints are sensitive.

Directions:

With your arms bent and your hands together and out in front of you, lower into a squat position.

Push through and land back on the balls of your feet after exploding up into a jump.

Squat down again when you reach the ground again, and do it again.

Perform 10-12 reps in three sets.

6. Burpees are another high-impact plyometric exercise that

targets the whole body and burns calories quickly.

Directions:

Start by standing straight, with your arms at your sides and feet shoulder-width apart.

Move your hands in front of you as you begin to squat. Extend your legs straight back as soon as they reach the ground so that you end up in a high plank position.

Jump your feet up to your palms by hinging at your waist as soon as you reach the high plank position. If necessary, place your feet outside of your hands and get as close to your hands as you can.

Jump squat immediately after getting up.

Extend your legs once more out after you land, and continue with steps 3–4.

Begin with 15 sets.

7. Standing side hops Lateral (side-to-side) exercises are an essential part of a comprehensive exercise program. Standing side hops improve ankle and hip mobility.

Directions:

Begin standing with your feet together and your arms at your sides bent at a 90-degree angle. Your knees ought to be supple.

Jump to the right while keeping your feet together, taking off, and landing on your heels.

Jump back to the left as soon as you get to the ground.

For three sets, perform 20 reps.

8. Pullups A standard pull-up is hard to do, even for people who exercise a lot. But the reward is worth it. You can still benefit from using a pull-up band for support.

Directions: Grip a pullup bar by standing underneath it and placing your hands slightly wider than shoulder-width apart.

Pull yourself up by bending your arms and pulling your elbows toward the ground after raising your feet off the ground and hanging from your arms.

9. Split squats Any exercise that targets your hamstrings, quadriceps, and glutes—your body's largest muscles—will pay big dividends. That's all there is to split squats.

Directions: Make a staggered stance by taking a large step forward with your left foot. Make sure you put equal weight on each foot.

Lower your body until your left knee is at a 90-degree angle by bending your knees.

Repeat the push-up exercise 12 times. Repeat with the other legs.

How exercise improves mental health

Exercise has also been found to alleviate symptoms such as low self-esteem and social withdrawal.3 Exercise is especially important in patients with schizophrenia because these patients are already vulnerable to obesity and also because of the additional risk of weight gain associated with antipsychotic treatment, particularly with atypical antipsychotics. Exercise improves mental health by reducing anxiety, depression, and negative mood as well as by improving self-esteem and cognitive function2. Thirty minutes of moderate exercises, such as brisk walking three days a week, is sufficient for these health benefits for schizophrenia patients who participated in a physical conditioning program for three months. These patients reported improved weight control, increased fitness, exercise tolerance, reduced blood pressure, increased perceived energy, and increased upper body and hand grip strength.5 In addition, these thirty minutes need not be continuous; It is believed that three 10-minute walks are just as beneficial as one 30-minute walk.

The following are some of the health benefits of regular exercise that every mental health professional should emphasize to their patients:

better sleep.

increased fascination with sex.

Enhancement of endurance

Stress relief

mood improvement.
increased power and endurance.
reduced fatigue that can lead to increased mental acuity.
lowering of weight.
lowered cholesterol and increased fitness in the heart.
Exercise is an essential part of changing one's lifestyle. Patients and mental health professionals alike do not adequately comprehend or appreciate the significance of exercise. Exercise may be a neglected mental health care

intervention, according to evidence.

Exercise reduces stress

When you exercise, your sense of well-being and overall health improve, giving you more energy every day. However, exercise also has some direct benefits for relieving stress.

1. It makes you feel good. Endorphins—the neurotransmitters in your brain that make you feel good—may increase when you exercise. Even though this state is often referred to as a runner's high,

it can be brought on by any aerobic activity, like a thrilling game of tennis or a hike through the woods.

2. It lessens stress's negative effects. While mimicking the effects of stress, such as the flight or fight response, exercise can help your body and its systems practice working together through those effects and relieve stress. Shielding your body from the negative effects of stress can also have beneficial effects on your cardiovascular,

digestive, and immune systems.

3. It's like moving meditation. You may frequently find that you have forgotten the problems of the day and are only focused on your body's movements after a fast-paced game of racquetball, a long walk or run, or several pool laps.

You may discover that focusing on a single task and the resulting energy and optimism can help you maintain calm, clarity, and focus in everything you do as you begin to regularly release your daily tensions through movement and physical activity.

4. It makes you feel better. Exercise on a regular basis can help you feel better, have a better mood, relax, and lessen the symptoms of mild depression and anxiety. Your sleep, which is frequently disrupted by stress, depression, and anxiety, can also be improved by exercise. All of these advantages of exercise can reduce stress

and give you a sense of control over your life and body.